The DASH Effect:

Instantly Return Your Body to Peak Physical Form

Aaron Holtz

Table of Contents

Introduction

The following chapters will discuss what the DASH Effect is and how it can transform your health. This book is not your typical 'get healthy now' book. It is not a book full of bland recipes. Nor is it a book that is preaching all the medical hype to you like your doctor would.

If you are nervous about starting a new diet and are not sure if the DASH Effect is right for you, then look no further. This is the book for you. It provides you a meal preparation worksheet along with a calorie tracker, and even a few recipes to show you how to incorporate the changes into your current cooking routine. There is no need to feel overwhelmed by the DASH Effect. It is not difficult to understand, and the benefits are amazing. Stop struggling with hypertension, diabetes, and depression. It is time to start eating healthier, and you can feel better knowing that you have control over managing your health.

By conducting extensive research, scientists have designed the DASH effect diet to help reduce hypertension, and through an amazing coincidence, they also discovered a way to reduce your insulin shot needs. But that's not all, they also helped you lose weight, fight cancer, osteoporosis, depression, heart disease, and diabetes all with this one clean eating diet.

If you think this is amazing, imagine what else it can do. But this is just the introduction, to get the full benefits of this book you must continue reading and start incorporating the DASH Effect into your life. To transform your health you must take action, and I think you already have a clue on what you need to do.

There are plenty of books on this subject on the market, so thanks again for choosing this one! Every effort was made to ensure that as much as possible the book is filled with plenty of useful information, please enjoy!

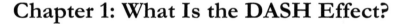

Chapter 1: What Is the DASH Effect?

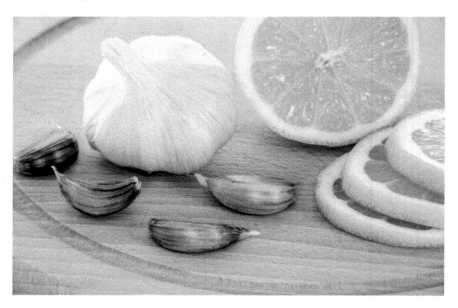

Are you suffering from hypertension? Do you need a great way to lower your sodium intake without losing the flavor in your meals? If you are searching for the most successful diet plan, then this is your book. The DASH effect diet was ranked the best diet for 7 years in a row by the United States News and World Report. If you've been looking for a weight loss program, then the DASH effect is exactly what you need.

The DASH effect diet is a diet designed to help reduce hypertension and lower blood pressure by providing a diet of clean, fresh foods with lots of color variety. By lowering your sodium intake, you can lower your blood pressure. It's also known to lower your blood sugar which makes it great for diabetics. So what is the DASH effect? Well, DASH is an acronym for 'Dietary Approaches to Stop Hypertension.' With many Americans suffering from hypertension, having a healthy diet full of fresh, clean foods is something that everyone needs.

Since the DASH effect started, it has been making headlines. It is promoted by the National Heart, Lung and Blood Institute for hypertension and blood pressure. The USDA says that the DASH effect is the ideal plan for Americans, and the Kidney Foundation has endorsed it for people suffering from kidney disease. With endorsements like these, why is everyone not following the DASH effect diet plan? The true answer is that change is hard. But the DASH effect diet doesn't have to be.

So what exactly is the DASH effect and how can you incorporate it into your life? Well, that is really quite easy. Since most of you are already eating the key foods in the DASH effect, it should not be much of a drastic change. I think the biggest change is the lower sodium intake. You see, in a normal American diet, we consume around 3,500mg of sodium per day. In the DASH effect diet plan, we want to lower our sodium intake. So why should we do that? Lowering our sodium intake to either 2,300mg per day or 1,500mg per day can make changes that will transform our health.

By lowering our sodium we can remedy our hypertension, also known as 'blood pressure,' and even reduce our systolic blood pressure. But that isn't all, we can also reduce blood sugar levels, and it aids in preventing osteoporosis, cancer, stroke, and diabetes. The added reward is by reducing our sodium intake and eating a cleaner more natural diet we are also reducing our caloric intake and thus by reducing our weight. Even though weight loss is not the reason for this dietary plan, it is an added benefit. Everyone is interested in losing weight and with the DASH effect diet you can do just that without missing out on caffeine, alcohol, sweets, fruits, vegetables, dairy, grains, or even dairy.

How do we do this? Well, it is as simple as portion control and choosing the proper ingredients for our meals. For instance, if you're having breakfast you would have:

- One store-bought, whole-wheat bagel with two tablespoons of peanut butter, without added salt of course

- 1 medium orange

- One cup of low-fat milk or lactose-free milk

- And 1 cup of decaffeinated coffee, without the sugar and cream

In the example above, not only do you have your wheat on your bagel, but you also have your protein in your peanut butter along with your coffee, dairy, and a fruit. Having this combination for breakfast will fill you up for the day while lowering your blood pressure. Each of these items is low in sodium, high in potassium, magnesium, and calcium. This breakfast gives you grains, fruit, dairy, and protein you'll need to start the day as recommended by the DASH effect diet meal plan. The best part about the DASH Effect is that you still get to have your caffeine, which helps boost your energy for the day ahead. This breakfast will provide you with the necessary nutrients that are needed to start your day on a healthy note.

The DASH effect is not like any other diet that you may have heard of. For instance, you do not have to eliminate your favorite foods. You just have to make a smarter choice when purchasing or preparing those foods. The DASH effect diet plan is so rich in potassium, magnesium, and calcium it provides a stronger foundation for your 2,000 calories nutritional intake that is recommended by the USDA for the average person. If you need a higher calorie diet, you can increase the intake of vegetables, fruits, and proteins to build a healthier balanced diet and still follow the DASH effect program.

So, "What can I eat in the DASH effect plan?" you may be asking. Well, you might be surprised to find that you can eat almost everything you already eat. It's a cleaner dietary plan with many great meal prep options that we will discuss later in this book. The DASH effect diet plan offers items such as fresh, clean, low-fat, and not processed foods. For example, you can eat fruits, vegetables, low-fat dairy, whole grains, fish, poultry, and nuts. In limited quantities, you can have beef, sweets, and sugary beverages. Caffeine and alcohol are not included in this meal plan. However, you can follow the USDA recommendation of an intake of no more than 2 alcoholic or caffeinated beverages for males per day, and no more than 1 alcoholic or caffeinated beverage for women per day. With caffeine, it is best to switch to decaffeinated beverages and eliminate the sugar and heavy cream. However, if you do have sugar in your coffee or heavy cream, you want to deduct that from your permissible caloric intake per day.

So what exactly are your permissible servings per day with the DASH effect meal plan for each food item? Let's start with your grains. You are allowed 7-8 grains per day. One serving of grains is equivalent to one slice of bread or 0.50 cup of pasta or rice. This is based on a 2,000-calorie diet per day. If you need a higher calorie intake diet, then it is suggested you do not add more grains to your servings intake, instead add more fruit or vegetables.

Your allowable vegetable servings per day are 4-5 servings. Suggested vegetables range from broccoli, carrots, tomatoes, sweet potatoes, Brussels sprouts, and other greens. A serving size is one cup of raw salad greens or a 0.50 cup of chopped vegetables. Your vegetable intake can be cooked or raw. You can use frozen or fresh vegetables. You can also have stir fry or à la carte vegetables. Adding a few extra vegetables to your meals is recommended instead of adding sweets or grains.

Fruit is another recommended dietary choice. You can have 4-5 servings of fruit per day. These servings can consist of bananas, apples, grapes, berries, and more. A medium sized fruit or 0.50 cup of fresh or frozen fruit is the suggested serving size. Fruits are a great way to have a light snack throughout the day. They also provide necessary natural sugars to your diet. Just make sure you follow the serving suggestions for snacks and meals.

Dairy is something we all struggle with. We either can't stomach it, or we drink too much heavy creams and whole milk. On the DASH effect diet plan, we can have low-fat or fat-free dairy products. These can be milk, yogurt, cheese, and other dairy items. We should have no more than 2-3 servings of dairy per day. Lactose-free products are listed within this category as well. Each serving size should be no more than one cup of milk or yogurt per serving.

If you choose to incorporate meat into your DASH food prep, then consider that you should have no more than six servings of meat per day. Each serving is 1 ounce. In most diets, we should only eat about two 3-ounce servings of meat a week. A standard deck of cards or the area of the palm of your hand is about 3 ounces of meat. It is best to have only grilled, baked, or broiled meats. Your meat choices should consist of lean ground beef, salmon, turkey, tuna, and chicken. Tuna and salmon are high in omega-3 fatty acids and helps lower cholesterol. Meat is not a required item for the DASH effect diet, so whether you add meat or not is a choice you will have to make.

Supplementing meat with legumes is perfectly fine as well. Legumes fall in the seeds category and no more than 4-5 servings per day should be consumed. These are almonds, sunflower seeds, kidney beans, peas, lentils, and other beans and nut seeds that are high in omega-3 fatty acids and monounsaturated fat. They are great to sprinkle on salads, stir-fry, and add a nice crunch to any meal. One nut to stay away from is coconuts, they do not provide the proper nutrients that you would need for this plan. A serving size for legumes is two tablespoons of sunflower seeds or 0.33 cup of nuts or beans.

You are allowed at least 2-3 servings of fats and oils per day on the DASH effect diet plan. Oils such as olive oil, margarine, and low-fat mayonnaise are all allowable oils for condiments and adding flavor. One serving size is one tablespoon of soft margarine or mayonnaise.

Although we should all avoid sweets and sugar since they add fat to our bodies, on the DASH effect diet plan there is room for five or fewer servings of sweets per week. Allowable sugars are jelly, sorbet, hard candies, and more. A serving size is one tablespoon of sugar or 0.50 cup sorbet. When adding these in try to find low-fat or fat-free options. Even low-fat cookies are a great option for you, just remember to keep track of any other ingredients that were added to the cookies like nuts.

If you are like most people, you start your day with a cup of coffee with cream and sugar. Even though these things can cause the inflammation of your body, they are allowed in the DASH effect diet plan. Men should not have more than 2 drinks per day of either coffee or alcohol, and women should have no more than 1 drink of coffee or alcohol. This is another great advantage to this dietary plan. So if you are a heavy coffee drinker, or if you love that glass of wine at night before bed, this is where the struggle might come in. By limiting the intake of these drinks, we will feel healthier, and our blood sugar will be lowered drastically as well as limit the inflammatory effects of caffeine on our body.

Why does it work?

Through extensive research and open trials conducted by the National Institute of Health, the data collected showed the patients with hypertension, high blood pressure, and diabetes experienced a decrease of symptoms while they were on the DASH effect diet plan. By gradually changing your eating habits to follow the DASH effect diet plan you are reducing your sodium intake and allowing your body to start healing. Start with one day a week and gradually work to a full week of eating healthy.

By changing your meal prep and choices for each meal, including snacks, you can gradually move up a day until you have fully integrated the DASH effect plan for every meal, seven days a week. Eliminate the sodium by not adding any more sodium to your meal prep and using an option for your foods that have a lower sodium content. A tablespoon of salt is equivalent to 2,325mg of sodium. The average person takes in 3,500mg per day. That is 1,200mg more than the standard DASH Effect plan and 2,000mg more than the lower sodium DASH plan. Preparing your meals with herbs and seasoning that have no added sodium will greatly reduce your sodium intake and aid in reducing those numbers drastically.

If your body has less sodium in it, your blood pressure drops, you start to feel better, and you can reduce your systolic blood pressure, giving you a better chance of not having a heart attack. A heart attack is one of the leading causes of death in the United States. Hypertension or high blood pressure is found in an average of 50 million people who have adhered to the American diet. That makes it about 1 billion people all over the world who are dealing with hypertension. That is why the DASH effect diet is recommended for all.

By eating foods high in potassium, magnesium, and calcium, we are lowering our blood pressure. The DASH effect is a dietary pattern, rather than a single nutrient diet, that's rich in antioxidants. It provides alternatives to junk food and eliminates the need for processed foods. By following a diet plan where you lower your sodium intake but increase your consumption of potassium, you are getting full and staying full longer allowing for fewer intakes of calories per day.

With the DASH effect diet plan, you will surely have a healthier body, and you will reduce your need for medication to control your blood pressure. It has also been shown that people who have participated in the studies exhibited signs of reduced depression. If we are happy with our health, we tend to be happier with our lives. By healing our bodies, we can heal our minds and feel like we can take on whatever life throws at us. So how do we follow this diet in our daily meal prep?

One way to follow this amazing diet plan is to ensure you have plenty of variety on the plate, you must have fruits, vegetables, and non-fat to low-fat dairy. With each meal, you should have two side dishes of vegetables and fruit-based desserts instead of desserts rich in sugar. You are eliminating the need for artificial sugars and processed foods. Reading labels before buying food helps us ensure we are buying the right ingredients and nutritional needs. We will discuss what we truly need later on in this book. For now, just know that reading labels and buying more fresh or frozen food options is our best way to ensure we are following the recommended food list.

In a typical DASH Effect daily meal plan, our nutritional values can look like this:

- Calories 2015

- Total fat 70g

- Saturated fat 10g

- Trans fat 0g

- Monounsaturated fat 25g

- Potassium 3,274mg

- Calcium 1,298mg

- Cholesterol 70 mg

- Sodium 1,607mg

- Total Carbohydrates 267g

- Dietary fiber 39g

- Total sugar 109g

- Protein 90g

- Magnesium 394mg

As you can see, the amount of sodium, sugar, saturated fat, and trans fat is reduced while the amount of potassium, magnesium, and calcium is increased, providing a better diet rich in nutrients. This is how we can lower our blood pressure, decrease our blood sugar, enhance the functions of our kidney, so we can feel healthier, alert, and energized.

Chapter 2: The Key Concepts Behind the DASH Effect

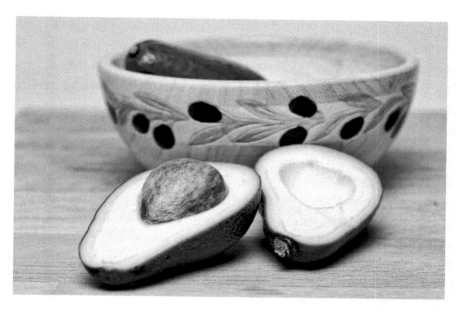

The DASH effect diet is a therapeutic approach to eating healthier. It helps you manage your weight, your blood pressure, your insulin sensitivity, and your blood cholesterol. What really makes the DASH effect diet great is that it not only lowers the blood pressure but it also, over time, helps you reduce your reliance on chemical substances. It is recommended for everyone from children to seniors who are trying to live healthy as much as possible. Not only does it provide health benefits, but it also has added benefit of helping you lose weight. There are no expensive supplements or shakes to purchase, making it a budget-friendly option for people who have limited funds. By eliminating processed foods, high sodium foods, all the fat in dairy, and lowering your intake of red meats, it also provides you with a low-sodium meal plan that will drastically reduce your risks of being afflicted with heart disease and cancer as well as diabetes and depression.

As with any diet or meal prep plan, there are key factors that determine why we need to change our eating habits. Whether it is high blood pressure or finding a healthier weight loss program, changing your dietary intake is hard. We don't make decisions to change our eating habits because we are told to by our doctors, it's not because the hottest stars are doing it, and it's not because we see our best friend or others online getting healthier either. It's because you are dealing with illness and want a better way to handle it, it is because you are ready to change your life and health.

When you get to the point that you have had enough of the pain, enough of the suffering from high blood pressure, enough of multiple prescriptions and are ready to make a difference in your life and your family's lives, that is when we start thinking about changing. By adding the DASH effect diet to our meal prep plans, we can start making those changes with minimal discomfort or inconvenience.

One thing we must be prepared to do is accepting that we no longer need the sodium and that food will taste good without it. Just give it time. After you eliminate all the sodium you have been adding to your meals, you will start to feel better, and your health will improve. You will notice that the taste of food has changed, and you will be able to taste more of the food and less of the sodium. Once you start the elimination process, you may feel as if your food has lost its flavor, but it hasn't. That is just the sodium leaving your body. Your taste buds will adjust themselves. Over time, you will start to taste the food, and you will have a deeper understanding of how your food should taste. You will have less of a craving for sodium, and you will even be able to tell if extra sodium was added to your food.

The key factor to making this change, and sticking with it, is to gradually reduce your sodium. Start with buying foods with low-sodium content and only sprinkling salt on the food while it cooks. Use a specific measurement and don't add any more after it is done. Gradually eliminate this habit of sprinkling salt and get used to the natural sodium that's in your food. As you decrease your sodium intake, you will notice your taste buds adjusting, and you will no longer need the sodium that you used to put on your food. The same goes for sugar and other things that you need to adjust to this diet.

By adding more fruit and vegetables to your meals, you are essentially getting those natural sugars that are necessary for your dietary and nutritional needs. Everything we eat has natural sugars, as young children we learn that sugar is good. However, we are not told that sugar can be found naturally in fruits and vegetables. As we get older, we struggle to let go of the sugars that we have added to our diet. Those sugars cause fat to build up in our bodies and can result in a higher risk of diabetes. Salt and sugar are among the hardest things to let go of, but it can happen.

If we eat healthier, we become healthier and more energized. Sugar and salt weigh us down and even make us look bloated. This can make us less energized and uncomfortable in our clothes. It increases our heart rate and changes the chemistry in our bodies. When we become healthier, our moods change, we can think better, and we won't have as many health issues. These are the key concepts behind the DASH effect diet plan.

Dietary recommendations with nutritional facts

A few dietary recommendations can make a world of difference as we transition to a new meal prep plan. What you should start with is some general knowledge about what nutrients are found in our foods. For example, fruits are low fast-food items with low sodium and lower cholesterol. This makes them a great source of vitamin C, folic acid, and dietary fiber. Fruits that are high in potassium are bananas, cantaloupe, dried apricots, and orange juice. Dietary fiber is found in fruits and can help reduce heart disease and helps with fiber intake which aids in bowel functions. Whole fruits contain enough dietary fiber to make you feel full, so you will only require a minimum amount of calories. Vitamin C helps repair body tissue and is necessary to maintain healthy teeth and gums.

Several vegetables have zero sodium content. Asparagus is one of these vegetables. If you add 5 spears of asparagus to a meal, that's enough to significantly reduce your sodium intake. Other zero-sodium vegetables are ⅓ portion of a medium cucumber, ¾ cups of green snap peas, ½ medium summer squash and 1 medium sweet corn ear. Try incorporating these into your meal prep plans. Every meal should have 1-2 vegetables. So think about adding in several more choices to your dinner plate.

Tilapia, tuna, salmon, catfish, and halibut all have low-sodium content. With a serving size of 3 ounces, you can incorporate either one of these fish into just about every meal. For example, you can have poached salmon and eggs for breakfast. Add in a cup of decaffeinated coffee and a slice of whole-wheat bread with light margarine and a medium apple, and you have yourself a very hearty breakfast with low sodium and a minimal number of processed foods. In this chapter, I have included several recipes and nutritional facts to help you start the DASH effect diet on your own.

The dietary needs of everyone and every age is different so following the standard 2000 calorie diet may not be the ideal diet plan for everyone. So I have included a dietary recommendation for women and men based on age groups below.

Age (Women)	Sedentary lifestyle	Moderate lifestyle	Active lifestyle
19-30	2000	2000-2200	2400
31-50	1800	2000	2200
51+	1600	1800	2000-2200
Age (Men)			
19-30	2400	2600-2800	3000
31-50	2200	2400-2600	2800-3000
51+	2000	2200-2400	2400-2800

Using these dietary daily nutritional values, we can then design a meal plan that incorporates these needs into the total calorie intake for the day. Below are a few recipes for meal prep items that can be used with fruit, grain, low-fat dairy, meat, and nuts or seeds of your choice. I started with a couple of breakfast recipes then provided you with a couple of lunch recipes as well as a couple of dinner recipes. Each recipe is designed to follow the DASH effect diet and is just a piece of the menu. You will notice that I have included alternatives to traditional flour as well as a vegan alternative for those who do not eat meats. Each recipe also indicates the nutritional value. Some of these recipes provide recommended toppings or garnish, and some of them are great to bring along to work as a snack or lunch.

Recipes for breakfast

Banana Pancakes

If you love bananas, then you are going to love these pancakes. This recipe should make about 4-6 pancakes and takes roughly 30-40 minutes to prepare.

Nutrition per serving:
- Calories 146
- Fat 4g
- Carbohydrates 22g
- Protein 7g
- Sodium 331g

What to use:
- Low-fat milk or lactose-free milk (0.33 cup)
- Chopped walnuts (1 tablespoon)
- Vanilla extract (0.50 teaspoon)
- Olive oil (1.50 teaspoon)
- Cinnamon (A small pinch)
- Salt (A small pinch)
- Large Eggs (2)
- Baking powder (1.0 teaspoon)
- Whole-wheat flour or coconut flour (0.33 cup)
- Mashed Banana (1)

What to do:
1. In a mixing bowl, combine all of the dry ingredients.
2. Separate the two eggs but keep the egg whites
3. In another mixing bowl, add olive oil, low-fat milk, egg whites, mashed banana, and vanilla until it's blended together well.

4. Combine the dry ingredients with the liquid ingredients. Using a spoon, stir until it's smooth.

5. Heat a griddle or frying pan over medium heat and apply a lite coating of olive oil to prevent the mixture from sticking. Place ¼ cup of the pancake mixture into a pan.

6. When you see bubbles around the edges of the pancakes, flip them over and continue cooking until the other side is done.

7. Sprinkle the chopped walnuts on top for added protein and texture.

Toppings:

- Sugar-free syrup
- Non-fat vanilla yogurt

Homemade Granola

This recipe takes 10 minutes to prepare, 30 minutes to cook, and makes 16 servings.

Nutrition per serving:
- Calories 199
- Fat 13g
- Sodium 86mg
- Carbohydrates 16g
- Protein 5g

What to use:
- Olive oil or Coconut oil (0.33 cup)
- Honey or Maple Syrup (0.33 cup)
- Salt (0.50 teaspoon)
- Cinnamon (2 Teaspoons)
- Protein Powder (0.50 cup)
- Flaxseed meal (0.50 cup)
- Raw pumpkin seeds (0.50 cup)
- Chopped walnuts (1 cup)
- Oats (2 cups)

What to do:
1. Start with preheating your oven to 325 °F.
2. Combine oats, walnuts, pumpkin seeds, flax, protein powder, cinnamon, and salt in a large mixing bowl.
3. Once everything is mixed well, drizzle with honey and then olive oil.
4. Stir until the mixture is evenly coated with both.
5. Prepare a baking sheet with wax paper.
6. Spread the mixture over the wax paper.
7. Continue to bake at 325°F for 30 minutes until golden brown.
8. Once done remove the granola from the stove and let it cool in the fridge for 2 hours.

Recipes for lunch

Spicy Peanut Tofu, Rice, and Avocado Salad

This recipe needs about 15 minutes to prepare. Serving size of 2 entrée sized salads.

Nutrition per serving:
- Calories 380 kcal
- Fat 18g
- Carbohydrates 42g
- Protein 15g
- Iron 14%
- Calcium 16%
- Vitamin A 15%
- Vitamin C 12%

What to use:
Dressing:
- Cayenne pepper (3-4 Dashes)
- Tamari (2 teaspoons)
- Water (0.50 cup)
- Agave syrup or Maple syrup (2 teaspoons)
- White miso paste (1 tablespoon)
- Peanut butter (2 tablespoons)

Salad:
- Mixed Spring greens (5 cups)
- Avocado, sliced-lengthwise (0.50 cups)
- Firm tofu, chilled and cubed (0.50 cup)
- Cooked brown rice (1 cup)

Garnish:
- Chopped cilantro

- Chopped peanuts
- Pepper or cayenne sprinkled on top (dash)

What to do:

1. Prepare your food processor or Vitamix.
2. Combine all the ingredients for the dressing in the food processor or Vitamix.
3. Blend until it's smooth and adjust the peanut butter as needed to get the richness of the sauce you wish for.
4. Prepare a pot with water and a pinch of salt. Once boiled, add the rice.
5. Cook rice until tender and done.
6. On a cutting board, dice up your tofu.
7. Toss your tofu in with the rice.
8. Add in a few spoonfuls of peanut sauce then proceed to toss the salad.
9. Place greens in a serving bowl.
10. Place sliced avocado over the top of the greens.
11. Decorating in a twirl design.
12. Place a scoop of the peanut tofu on top of the salad.
13. Add more dressing as needed, plus the cilantro and peanuts, cayenne pepper.

Poppy Seed Chicken Noodle Casserole

This is a twist on the classic chicken casserole. It takes 50 minutes to bake chicken and up to 2 hours once it's placed in the slow cooker.Serving size is 4.

Nutrition per serving:
- Calories 411.3
- Total Fat 8.1 g
- Cholesterol 68.4 mg
- Sodium 251.8 mg
- Carbohydrates 47.4 g
- Protein 38.7 g

What to use:
- Light buttery spread (4 tablespoons)
- Poppy seed (2 Teaspoons)
- Frozen peas (2 cups Thawed)
- Whole-wheat pasta (4 cups)
- Boneless and skinless chicken breast (2)

What to do:
1. Preheat oven to 325 °F.
2. Once it's preheated, place the chicken in a pan and cook.
3. While cooking chicken, cook the pasta until it's tender.
4. Once the pasta is done, place it in the slow cooker on low temperature.
5. Add the peas.
6. Add the poppy seeds.
7. Add the buttery spread.
8. Once the chicken is done, add it too.
9. Cook in the slow cooker until the peas are warm or for 30 minutes minimum or 2 hours maximum.
10. Season to taste.

Recipes for dinner

Easy Sweet Potato Veggie Burgers, with Avocado

This is a vegan twist on the traditional burger. Who says burgers can't be vegan?

This recipe makes 6-8 burgers and takes 10 minutes to prepare and 80 minutes to cook.

Nutrition per serving:
- Total carbohydrates: 30g
- Protein: 7g
- Fat: 4g
- Calories: 176g
- Dietary fiber: 5g

What to use:
- Chopped greens (kale, spinach, parsley) (0.33-1 cup finely)
- Nutritional yeast or any flour (try oat flour) (0.33 cup)
- Black pepper (add more for more bite!) (0.25 teaspoon)
- Salt (0.50 teaspoon)
- Chipotle powder or Cajun spice (use more for spicier burgers, (0.50 -1 teaspoon)
- Garlic powder (1 teaspoon)
- Apple cider vinegar (0.75 teaspoon)
- Tahini (2-3 tablespoons)
- White onion, chopped (0.50 cup)
- Cooked white beans (canned, drained and rinsed) (16 ounces)
- Sweet potato, baked and peeled (1 medium)

Toppings:
- Avocado, tomato, Vegenaise, burger buns, greens

Skillet:
- Virgin coconut oil (1 tablespoon)

Optional:
- Panko breadcrumbs for crispy coating

What to do:
1. Preheat oven to 400 °F.
2. Bake the potato for 40-60 minutes or until tender.
3. Combine potato and beans in a large mixing bowl. Beans must be rinsed before you add it to the bowl.
4. Using fork or masher, mash together the ingredients in the bowl.
5. Put in the white onions and keep mashing.
6. Put in the tahini, garlic, chipotle, salt and pepper, yeast, greens, and apple cider vinegar.
7. Keep on mashing until it's thoroughly mashed.
8. With the oven at 400 °F, heat a skillet on the stovetop over high heat and add the coconut oil.
9. Form burger patties and roll in panko crumbs if using them then place on the skillet to cook.
10. Cooking time is 1-3 minutes per side, cook patties until light brown.
11. Then repeat with all the rest of the patties, making around 6-8 patties.
12. Once all the patties are cooked, place them on a baking sheet lined with wax paper and bake for 10-15 minutes, cooking all the way through.
13. While baking the burgers, slice up your toppings for decorating the burgers.
14. Toast your whole-wheat bun in a toaster (any whole-wheat, high-fiber bun will work).
15. Add vegan mayonnaise and spicy mustard to the bun

16. When burgers are done add burger to bun and the top with your choice of toppings.
17. Serve warm!

Note: You can store the remaining burgers in a sealed container in the fridge for a day or freezer for a week. You just have to reheat it at 400 °F for about 12 minutes.

Easy Roasted Salmon

This is part of a dinner dish that includes roasted salmon. Also, you will add vegetables and fruit along with some grain. This recipe takes 10 minutes to prepare and 22 minutes to cook. Serving size of 4.

Nutrition per serving:
- Sodium 78 mg
- Calories 251
- Potassium 894 mg
- Calcium 36 mg
- Cholesterol 94 mg
- Carbohydrates 2 g
- Fat 11g
- Magnesium 53 mg
- Saturated Fat 2g
- Dietary Fiber less than 1 g
- Sugars less than 1 g
- Protein 34g

What to use:
- Garlic cloves, minced and peeled (4)
- Fresh ground pepper
- Lemon, cut (4 wedges)
- Minced fresh dill, from one small bunch (0.25 cup)
- Wild salmon fillets (4-6 ounce pieces)

What to do:
1. Preheat oven to 400 °F before starting.
2. Bring out a glass baking dish and coat it with coconut oil.
3. Place your salmon fillets in the dish.

4. Using the 4 wedges of lemon, squeeze one per fillet on top of the fillets.
5. Then sprinkle black pepper, garlic, and dill on each fillet.
6. Bake for 20-22 minutes until the fillets are opaque in the center.

Chocolate Banana Cake

This is a blend of chocolate and banana which blends really well with the cake texture. The preparation time is about 15 minutes and cooking time is around 25 minutes. This recipe can make around 18 servings.

Nutrition per serving:
- Calories: 150
- Sodium: 52 milligrams
- Potassium: 119 milligrams
- Magnesium: 19 milligrams

What to use:
- Large egg (1)
- Canola oil (0.25 cup)
- Soy milk (0.75 cup)
- Ripe banana, mashed (1 large, 0.50 cup)
- Baking soda (0.50 teaspoon)
- Splenda brown sugar blend (0.50 cup)
- Unsweetened cocoa powder (0.25 cup)
- Semisweet dark chocolate chips (0.50 cup)
- All-purpose flour (2 cups)
- Vanilla extract (1 teaspoon)
- Egg white (1)
- Lemon juice (1 tablespoon)

What to do:
1. Preheat your oven to 350 °F.
2. Using olive oil, coat a nonstick brownie pan.
3. Add flour to a bowl.
4. Blend in the brown sugar.
5. Cocoa and baking soda.

6. In a separate bowl throw in the bananas.
7. While whisking, pour in the soy milk, oil, eggs, egg whites, lemon juice, and the vanilla.
8. Once everything is blended, make a cavity in the flour and slowly pour in the liquid mix.
9. Add the chocolate chips.
10. Using a wooden spoon, stir to blend the ingredients.
11. Once it's thoroughly blended, spoon mixture into a brownie pan.
12. Bake for 25 minutes.
13. Take it out and use a toothpick to check the center if it is cooked all the way through.

Chapter 3: Why We Need the DASH Effect to Stay in Peak Form

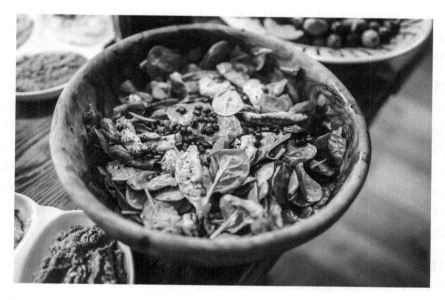

Now that you know a little bit more about the DASH effect diet and how it helps your body become healthier, let's discuss why you need the DASH effect and how the myths and negative misconceptions should not be an issue once you're on this meal plan.

As we grow up, our diets get discombobulated, and we start consuming too many fried foods, too much fat, heavy creams, and way more sugar and sodium than we should have ever consumed. There is no clear-cut reason why we do this. As we age, we start trying new things, and we find an easier way to prepare meals, and we all too often take the lazy choice of stopping at the local McDonald's. Through years of eating unhealthy foods, we developed high blood pressure, insulin spikes, heart conditions, diabetes, and even depression.

We don't consider that our diet is the main cause, so we go to the doctor and get medicine that is designed with chemicals, similar to the processed foods that we have been consuming for years. The medicines help, but they do not eliminate the problem, in fact, they increase our need to be dependent on chemical-based foods and medicine. So what do we do about it? We continue to eat the garbage that is killing us, and we wonder why we aren't getting any better.

This is a cycle of self-destruction that we have carried from the early stages of life where we learned our eating habits and developed a taste for food. The DASH effect diet is against what we know as the normal way to enjoy our foods. It scares people to think that lower sodium could actually transform their health. If you are anything like the average American, you probably didn't realize the amount of sodium that is in your standard everyday diet.

That is why the DASH effect diet is the ideal way to get your health back on track. We don't need added salt in our foods. We don't need to consume 66 pounds of sugar per year. We definitely don't need to be dependent on chemical-based food and drinks. So how do we change this? We follow the DASH effect diet.

If you have been following me up until now, then you know that there are many benefits you can gain from following the DASH effect diet, and you are probably considering changing your eating habits. Maybe you're a little hesitant about eliminating the sugar and salt in your diet. You probably think that your food will not taste as good. Maybe you have tried other diets in the past, but you always ended up falling back on your old eating patterns.

Well, the good thing about the DASH effect diet is that it isn't like any other diet on the market. That is because it isn't a diet plan at all. It is a complete change in your eating patterns. But you don't have to actually change much of what you are already doing. It's mostly about portion control and buying cleaner and fresher ingredients.

If you are part of the meat-eating community that consumes 52.2 million pounds of meat per year, then it may be a bit difficult to alter your meat options for a while. In the DASH effect plan, you eat less red meat and more poultry, fish, and turkey. These are leaner meats with less fat and cholesterol. They also have a lower sodium content than pork and beef. If you are not a meat eater, then this diet will be an easy change for you. Many of the recipes that are available on the DASH effect diet are not only dairy-free but meat-free as well, making this a vegan-friendly diet.

Every year more and more people are being diagnosed with hypertension, diabetes, and heart disease. With the alarming numbers of people who suffer with these disorders, we need to consider why no one has changed their diet plan. Maybe it is out of fear of losing control over their food options. Maybe it is just because of plain stubborn behavior. Whatever the reason may be, Americans are not changing their eating patterns, it is clear that continuing the cycle of fat, deep fried, high-sodium meals are not doing any wonders for their health. The DASH effect is recommended not only by one scientist but by several companies and agencies who fight for a healthier America.

Why should you transition to the DASH effect diet? The answer: because it simply works. It's that simple and that easy. Scientifically, it has been proven to work. If something works as well as this does, it's a surprise that the school systems are not incorporating it into their weekly meal prepping for students.

How the benefits outweigh any myths or negative press on the effects

So why hasn't it taken off? There is a long-running myth that fresh foods are not as cheap as processed foods. But this simply isn't true. The process of preparing fresher foods that are richer in vitamins and nutrients and contain less fat-burning calories means that you will need a lower intake of calories and that your food will keep you full longer, essentially costing less in the long run.

People often believe that going to the drive-thru at McDonald's or Burger King is easier than preparing a kale salad. After a long day at work, you don't feel like coming home to prepare a healthy meal. It takes longer, and you just don't have the time or energy. This too is not true. It takes about 15 minutes to prepare a meal acceptable for the DASH effect diet, once all the prep work has been completed. You can also prepackage your ingredients or practice food prep procedures by preparing your ingredients before work and placing them in a slow cooker to simmer all day. This allows for you to simply come home, grab a bowl, and relax on the couch or at the table with family while enjoying a healthy, clean, and fresh meal.

Many people believe that there is a learning curve to proper nutritional calorie intake food prep. This as well is not true. There are so many recipes and cookbooks on the market that are geared towards healthier and cleaner eating that you'll find a recipe in no time to prepare for dinner. The best part is whatever you have left over from dinner can be utilized for breakfast or even lunch depending on what it is. Many of our food options on the DASH effect diet plan can be used for multiple meals, such as apples can be used as breakfast, fruit side dishes, and even desserts.

Often times, people think that eating healthy means eating bland food. That simply isn't true. Just because it's healthy doesn't make it bland. There are so many reasons why this myth is present, one of them being that throughout our life we have added salt and sugar to everything we eat, chose the fattest parts of the meat, and excessively flavored our foods. We do this because we are conditioned into thinking that we must add flavor to food. However, food already has a flavor. The natural juices and flavors that are ingrained in the fruit and vegetables provide all the flavor you need for your meal to taste amazing.

Now that doesn't mean that adding herbs to your food isn't a good thing. Many herbs and nectars provide healing benefits that just can't be ignored. Rosemary helps with immunity and honey is an antihistamine. Garlic is good for reducing blood pressure as well as combating the common cold. Sage is known for its anti-inflammatory properties as well as antioxidants. As you can see, many herbs and nectars provide added benefits to your food. So the best rule of thumb is to taste the natural foods then add in a few flavors through fresh herbs to give it an added health benefit.

Herbs can be purchased dried as well as fresh. Many people believe the benefits of herbs are just as effective when dried. I find that fresh herbs give a much better aromatic smell and tend to have a fresher, cleaner taste. They blend better with our foods and gives that added touch of texture that you just can't get from powders or dried herbs. They also are not processed heavily and have not been mixed with added sodium and other chemicals to make them last longer. As with any fresh food, being frozen is the best route since they still retain all the nutrients that provide you with the healthiest caloric intake.

Many Americans have been buying processed and canned

foods since World War 2. They are marketed as containing all the health benefits of a fresh batch of vegetables. However, through the process of canning or processing at the factory, we have learned that they are missing key components to their nutritional value. So the myth that canned or processed foods are just as good as fresh is completely wrong. Not only are they higher in sodium, since it is added for flavor and sustainability. But they are having their key nutrients flash steamed or cooked out of them and then being mixed with sustainable chemicals to make them last longer on the shelf. Taking all this into account, we should always purchase our foods frozen or fresh to ensure we are feeding ourselves and our families the best possible combination of nutrients that we can afford. One way we can do this is through farmers' markets and at local farms.

Buying your food at a farmers' market or picking your own at a local farm can also reduce the cost of the food you are purchasing. Knowing what you want to prepare in advance is also a way of reducing your cost of groceries, and it will also provide you with a guideline to decide on what kind of meal you should cook each day. This allows you to prepare your ingredients in advance and be ready for mealtime without the extra hassle. It doesn't take a ton of extra time to learn how to prepare in advance. You simply need to know what you like and have a recipe or idea of how you want to prepare a meal once you're ready for meal prep time. This will cut down on the amount of time it takes to prepare the meal without adding extra time to your daily to-do list. Later in this book, we will lay out a method to meal prep with a list of options for each meal and a way to incorporate an accountability partner into your diet change.

Chapter 4: Who Should Not Use the DASH Effect and Why?

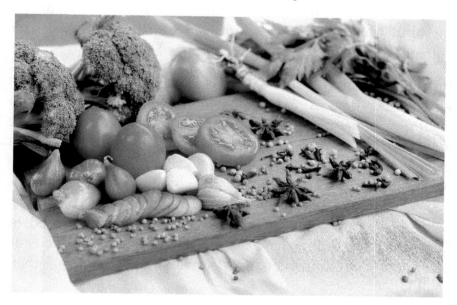

Previously, we discussed who the DASH Effect diet is ideal for. As rated by the Food and Drug Administration the DASH Effect diet is rated safe for everyone. So who shouldn't use the DASH effect diet then? Well, that is simple, this diet is not for people that are not committed to making a positive change in their lives. If you do not want to be healthier, if you do not want to lose weight, if you enjoy having diabetes and hypertension, if you do not want to transform your health and make changes to your lifestyle that will reduce your blood pressure, help you lose weight and also feel more happy in general about life, then you should not use the DASH effect diet.

Who in your family does this sound like? Is this person you? Or is it someone else that has been using their disease as a reason to play the victim every day of their life? You see the DASH effect diet is not for quitters. It's not for those people who love having sickness and struggle to keep up with their children or grandchildren. It is not for those that would rather eat a high-sodium and high-sugar diet. It is definitely not for those people who think that if their food is not loaded with bacon grease, it's not good.

In today's families, we all have that one person that doesn't watch what they eat. They think food doesn't determine their health, or they just really don't care. That person is not the ideal person to try the DASH effect diet. Not because they don't need it, not because it wouldn't help them, and definitely not because they are immune to its benefits or allergic to the process. No, those people are not ideal for the DASH effect diet because they do not care how they are treating their bodies. They don't care if they have ailments that they can reduce and eliminate. The simply do not care about the state of their health.

So how do you help those who don't care? We all would know they need the DASH effect diet and that if they were to give it a try, they would not only be happier, but they will also see drastic changes in their health for the better. So instead of shoving the DASH effect diet down their throats and trying to force them to get healthy, we must first get healthy ourselves. The best way to lead someone to a better path for their life is to show them through your own actions that it works and to essentially trigger their jealousy, so they want to get healthy to spite you.

Now I know this sounds a bit petty and far-fetched, but isn't it true that sometimes you only wanted something simply because someone else had it? Exactly, so now you see where this chapter is going. So far we have discussed what the DASH effect diet is, whom it's suited for, why it is effective, and now we will discuss the positive effects it has on our mental psyche.

Have you ever done something that you thought you were going to fail at, but in the end you actually did not fail? What about winning an award for something you did inadvertently while doing something else? Well, that feeling you got when that award was won, or that amazing realization that you actually succeeded instead of failing is what the DASH effect diet does for your psyche. Imagine going in for a haircut and coming out with a stylish haircut, a new dye job, and some free hair-conditioning supplies.

When you get so focused on creating a healthy eating habit you forget about so many other things that you are accomplishing. Such as losing weight or lowering your insulin injection needs. What if we could all just wake up with no depression, no diseases, no cancers, and no excess fat? With the DASH effect diet, we eventually can. Now, do you still want to question the validity of the DASH effects?

To get healthy and reduce your blood pressure you have to start somewhere, and the DASH effect diet is exactly where you need to start. Do not be disappointed if you have setbacks because they are normal. As long as you figure out the triggers and do what you can to avoid them you should be able to continue the program without too many setbacks.

But what if my blood pressure isn't elevated? Well, then the DASH effect diet is still the best for you. It is a starting point for a healthier and cleaner lifestyle. No, I don't mean cleaner like you cleaned your house. By saying cleaner, I mean that your food comes from the ground, with no pesticides, no growth hormones, no chemicals, and no processing.

What else do you need to know to understand that the DASH effect diet is for everyone? All it takes to find out if it is for you, besides me telling you it is, is to get started today. In this book, I have provided you a detailed description of what the DASH effect is and how to incorporate it into your life. But one thing we haven't talked about yet is the motivation you need to bring about changes in your life with the DASH effect. That is what this whole chapter will be on, motivational techniques to keep you focused, to keep you moving forward, and to show those stubborn family members who think that food does not heal, that in fact, it does.

One proven method to motivate you to continue on your journey with the DASH effect diet is to see progress. Progress is wonderful. It's like a reward in itself. When you see that your blood pressure is lower or you are experiencing less blood sugar spikes for example. That is called progress. Maybe your doctor has noticed a positive change in your blood. Maybe when you stand in front of the mirror after your shower, you see a slimmer and healthier you. Progress can be anything from a slight change in the size of your pants to a drastic drop in your need for your blood pressure medication. Whatever progress you achieved, regardless of how small it is, you need to celebrate.

Celebrate in ways that don't undermine your progress. There are many ways to celebrate your progress without having to derail your new lifestyle. One of my favorite ways to celebrate a positive change in my life is to immediately give myself praise. I look myself in the mirror, and I tell myself all the things that are wonderful about what I have accomplished. I acknowledge the efforts I have made, and I congratulate myself on a job well done. This is a personalized pat on the back.

Another way to reward yourself is to buy yourself a new piece of clothing, something that fits your new waistline. This tells your mind that you are making changes to get a more beneficial lifestyle. It also gives you a wonderful endorphin boost when you look at that new, slim piece of clothing and think, "I did this." Just remember that you are working towards a healthier you and that healthier 'you' will need a whole new wardrobe eventually. By throwing away clothes that no longer fit, you are subconsciously telling your mind and body that you will no longer accept what your body was back then. This is like a confirmation that you are a new person. Buying new clothes helps us physically see the changes we are making, giving us a good reason to celebrate our accomplishments and progress while making sure we look amazing.

Accountability is another great way to reward yourself when you see great progress. Accountability is when someone else will hold you accountable for your goals. This will be discussed later in Chapter 6, but for now, we will just state that accountability is calling your friend, your mom, or your exercise buddy and celebrating with them about your progress. Remember they are on your side and know that you need this healthier lifestyle.

There are so many ways to celebrate your achievements. By setting goals and reaching them, you are rewarding yourself every day when you pick healthier options and become a healthier you. Sometimes just knowing is enough of a reward. However, if knowing that you are getting healthier isn't enough, you can always try a day at the spa, a movie with your best friend, or even a night out with your favorite girl/guy.

One of the best rewards you can give yourself is acknowledging that you have done it on your own, without medicines, without surgeries, and without sitting around thinking there is nothing you can do to get healthier. You are the deciding factor, and you made that one decision to make your life better. Whatever you choose as a reward, make sure it is something that will give you excitement and that feeling of accomplishment. When we don't feel like we accomplished something big, we tend to feel more sad than happy. The trick is to be excited about your progress even if it seems insignificant.

Chapter 5: Specific Benefits to Your Health Gained from the DASH Effect

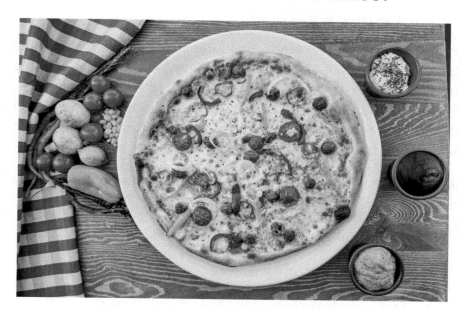

Since you made it this far, you have heard over and over that the DASH effect has outstanding scientific evidence showing its validity and the effects it has on your health. So what more can I say to motivate you on getting started with the DASH effect diet? Maybe with the amazing effects the DASH diet can have on our health, we will see a potential for lower insurance rates. Not only are our insurance rates on the verge of dropping because of this amazing diet, but it's also a national dietary method that's been recommended for over 10 years. Another benefit to the DASH effect diet is that previous studies proved that staying on the DASH effect diet can result in a reduction of systolic and diastolic blood pressure. These results were across all age groups, races, and genders. That means that this diet works for all races.

We all know that many African Americans suffer from race-specific anomalies and that these anomalies can cause certain diseases to be more dominant and prevalent. One thing scientists learned in the trials was that this diet worked amazingly on the African American community as well as the Caucasians, Asians, and Indians.

Further findings revealed that the DASH effect diet also lowered the risk of stroke and coronary heart disease, making it beneficial for people who are afflicted with such conditions. The DASH effect diet has also helped with bone loss and density, reducing bone turnover, which means an improvement in bone health for those prone to osteoporosis.

There are many ways for the DASH effect diet to help you with weight loss. Below are just a few of the ways:

- Fruits and veggies are low in calories.

- They are more filling as well

- You include protein-rich foods in every meal

- Using protein for snacks can increase your energy

- Protein makes meals more satisfying

- Protein also helps with in-between blood sugar crashes

- By focusing on the healthy foods, you eliminate the need for junk foods

- By eating denser foods, you reduce your cravings

- You can make the DASH effect diet your lifestyle diet plan

- It's not a fad diet

- Carbohydrates are not used to fill you up

- The plan doesn't limit your protein

- There is less starch

- Protein supports muscle mass

- Proteins are energy boosters and provide us the energy to exercise more efficiently

High blood pressure is a big reason why the DASH effect is popular. By reducing your sodium intake, you end up reducing your blood pressure. There are a few other benefits that we haven't discussed throughout this book:

- It helps reduce your blood pressure by reducing sodium in your diet

- It also helps by reducing your weight which can raise your blood pressure

- By reducing your weight and raising your protein intake you have more energy

- More energy means you can exercise more and help lower your blood pressure

- The DASH effect diet provides a healthy eating plan that not only reduces your blood pressure but helps keep it stabilized

We all know that high blood pressure increases the risk of getting heart disease and can contribute to several other diseases and ailments. The DASH effect can help eliminate the chances of heart disease by lowering your blood pressure. Several of the benefits of the DASH effect have been discussed throughout this book and in this chapter. But there are more benefits that the DASH effect can provide to aid in lowering the risk of heart disease:

- By adding more fiber, calcium, and magnesium, you can reduce the risk of heart disease

- Those three minerals help regulate blood pressure

- Potassium stops the effects of sodium

- The DASH effect diet is a sustainable diet, it is not something that will end immediately

- It's low in sodium and high in nutrient-rich foods

- It is adaptable, low stress, and easily customizable, making it the best diet choice for all

Even with all the benefits that the DASH effect diet has been proven to have on your health, not many people are using it. Though it has changed the way people think about eating and how food can transform your health, people are still so reluctant to what they have considered as proper eating their whole life. So why are more people not using the DASH effect diet? This is partly because the patients who need the diet the most are only getting medicinal help from their primary care providers. Not many doctors have nutritional backgrounds and lack knowledge in this area. Perhaps many people can be helped immensely if part of a doctor's training included nutrition and diet plans.

Although doctors are not trained to properly help those dealing with a diet issue, nutritionists are, and there are many ways you can get in contact with one. Health coaches are trained to help you find the right diet plan for your needs. Some of them should be listed in your local online business directory. Finding the right coach to help you with the DASH effect diet will take some time. Try asking family and friends. Get opinions online from trusted friends. Research the options in your area and know exactly what you are looking for.

Even with all the research and referrals, you still won't be able to know if that coach is right for you until you have a face-to-face meeting with them. So sit down with the coach of your choice and ask all the questions that you need to. Make sure you make a list of the questions you want to ask, this will ensure that you will get to know that person better. Once you run out of questions, ask the coach if there is anything else they would like to include in their comments or if they have any questions. This is a sure way to hear out your coach's opinions.

Remember they are the experts and know exactly what to do to help you with your dietary needs. One question you might ask is: "Are they familiar with the DASH effect diet?" This should instantly tell you whether or not they are the right nutritionist for you.

With all the talk about nutrition, food portions, and benefits associated with the DASH effect diet, this book would not be complete without helpful tools. These tools are designed to teach you how to incorporate proper meal preparations, exercise, accountability, and so much more. For the next chapter, we will be looking at those tools, and we will learn how to utilize them. The first tool we will look at is accountability, how you can find an accountability partner, and what you can expect from an accountability partner. You will notice that in this section we discussed nutritionists and health coaches a little bit more. That is because a health coach is a great accountability partner. Part of their roles in your life is to help you become accountable for your food choices, they act as your support system, and of course, they're your motivational coach.

The next part would deal with the subject of getting healthy with the help of exercise. We discussed various ways to incorporate exercise into your healthy lifestyle. There are many forms of exercise, and as a person with health issues, you might want to consult a doctor about appropriate exercises that you can do without endangering your health. Making sure that you are not overexerting yourself or injuring yourself is the best way to start a new exercise routine. In the next chapter, we will talk about yoga, running, jogging, and cardio. These are all acceptable exercises even for someone who has been dealing with various health concerns.

Meal prep is a big part of the DASH effect diet, and it can make or break your progress. Since you were proactive and bought this book, you have already set yourself up for success. This book not only explains the information on why this diet plan works, but it also helps you prepare the right meals so that you can take complete advantage of the DASH effect diet. Meal preparation is an easy thing to do if you use the worksheet provided in the next chapter. There is a designated section for each day and each meal. There is also a list of serving sizes and approved foods.

This is just a starting point. Once you get the hang of the process, you will find yourself creating your own meal preparation worksheets or even designing a digital one to use on the go. Meal preparation sounds like a chore, but you shouldn't feel discouraged because it can give you something to look forward to, such as that amazing meal you planned for the next day.

But meal preparations would be nothing without the calorie intake worksheet. It is designed to show you during the first few weeks of your journey into the DASH effect diet how well you are following the guidelines set by the program. By keeping track of the calories that you are taking in and making sure you stay within the recommended limits for each nutrient, you are following the program as designed. Doing what you can to meet the requirements of the DASH effect diet can help make sure that you will arrive at the desired outcome, a healthier and happier life.

Chapter 6: Ways to Include the DASH Effect into Your Daily Meals

There is so much information about the DASH effect diet packed into this book that I'm sure it is confusing, and you are probably feeling a bit overwhelmed. But there's no need to stress yourself out. We will now talk about how you can incorporate it into your daily meals.

We all hear that breakfast is the most important meal of the day, and if you are like most Americans, you either do not have time for breakfast or you just grab something from the local donut shop or McDonald's on the way to work. If you want to adhere to the principles of the DASH effect diet, that will not do. We are looking for cleaner, healthier ways to get all the nutrients we need for the day without all the added sodium and processed foods. So when we grab a donut from the local donut shop, we are basically fueling our day from the start with sugar, and that isn't good. When you start your day with sugar by mid-morning, you will have a sugar crash and need an energy boost later on. Instead, we should start the day with protein and low-sodium, low-sugar foods.

One of the best ways to start your day would be with a granola bowl packed with nuts, fruits, oats, and honey. This sounds like a lot of work, but it's really quite easy. You can prepare this in advance and have it stored in your fridge in mason jars so you can bring it to work. There are many recipes online that you can use, and many of them have nutritional information so you can track your calorie intake. You can use the worksheet which is found later in this book.

It isn't very hard to incorporate a new eating plan into your day, it just takes a bit of conscious effort to change the way you have been doing things. It can be scary but knowing that you are doing it to improve your health is a great way to keep you motivated as you continue your transition to a healthier life.

As you try to make your diet super healthy, you will notice that you are feeling more energized, and you will feel like you want to do more exercises during the day. Later in this chapter, we will discuss exercises that you can incorporate into your lifestyle to add to the DASH effect program and help you with establishing your healthier, new life. For now, just understand that if you have been sedentary for a while or if you are not as active as you should be, it will take time, and you should start slow, so you don't burn out quickly.

Accountability is another thing that will make this journey through the DASH effect program easier. Accountability is the number one thing that people who are making changes in their life say they lack. Many people aren't sure how to acquire an accountability partner nor are they sure about what one should be doing for them. Later on, we will discuss accountability and how it can help you with your healthier lifestyle journey.

This chapter is packed full of great resources and tools that will aid you in transforming your life with the help of the DASH effect diet. To make the most out of this book and the DASH effect you definitely need to use the information in this chapter to its fullest potential. By using all of these tools, you are giving yourself a greater advantage at accomplishing your goals such as seeing your blood pressure lower and a decrease in your medical expenses.

Exercise

Exercise is an integral part of your daily needs. If you are eating healthy and not doing any exercises, then you are only doing half the work. Starting an exercise routine when you feel like you have more energy is a great way to aid in your process of lowering your blood pressure. There are many exercise programs out there, and there are plenty of ways to incorporate them into your lifestyle. What you can start with is light cardio.

Cardio is any exercise that is mild and gets your heart rate up. You can start with walking at a fast pace. If you choose walking as an exercise, you should increase your heart rate just enough that you start breathing heavily, but you should still be capable of holding a conversation without gasping for air. Gasping for air means that you are overexerting your body and no longer burning calories. If you do incorporate a cardio routine into your lifestyle, make sure you increase your calorie intake based on the chart listed in chapter 2.

If cardio is not your style, a light yoga exercise is also a great way to stretch and get that heart rate up. Starting with the beginner's yoga, you can learn the proper techniques to doing yoga and increase your body's strength and flexibility. Yoga is incredibly beneficial to your body and your mind. Not only does it provide you a mindfulness exercise, but it helps you stretch those muscles that have been weighed down by the excess fat that you have been carrying. Yoga can be practiced at home with some really great YouTube yoga teachers, or you can get a membership to a Yoga studio and get personalized help with a custom muscle test and body flexibility test. As with any exercise program consult your doctor before starting.

If those two do not sound like your cup of tea then maybe you should try jogging, running, or weightlifting. Whatever it is that you end up picking, make sure you have consulted your doctor before starting a new exercise routine. As with any new activity or change in your life, there will be some difficulties, which is why you need to stay vigilant and determined to continue with making healthy changes in your life.

Accountability

Accountability is something we hear about often. When we are at work, we are accountable for our work and the work of our teams or employees. When we go to the gym, our spotter is accountable for our lives when we exercise. As we drive down the road, we are accountable for all the pedestrians, other cars, and people in our cars to keep them safe. So the concept of accountability is nothing new.

The difference between this accountability and the others listed above is that here we are having someone else help us be accountable for making positive changes in our lives. Maybe your doctor is your accountability partner, or maybe he or she is just monitoring your changes. If you have a strong partner who can help you through the process of change, then you should know what a strong support system feels like. However, if your partner is not very helpful or you are single, then you need to find someone to help you as an accountability partner.

One of the best ways to find an accountability partner is to find someone who is willing to help you make these positive changes in your life. Talk with your friends, your family, your workout buddies, maybe even your desk mate at work. Also, your partner must change as well if they need to. If you can't find anyone in your own group or circle, then check with a nutritionist that follows the DASH effect program and sign up for accountability partner programs. You can find these online.

A health coach is someone that will help you with your food choices and teach you how to bring the DASH effect diet off the road and into restaurants. They will also help you with grocery shopping. Sometimes we need that extra help so that we don't get overwhelmed. That is where the health coach comes in. They will hold you accountable when you need that extra kick to continue on your healthy journey. As an accountability partner, you can expect them to be vigilant with your progress. They will give you tasks to complete, and they will not allow you to fail. They will also be there to celebrate with you when you accomplish wonderful things through your lifestyle change.

Celebrating your accomplishments with someone is one of the perks of having a health coach. They get to see you go through your trials and tribulations. They get to watch you succeed and see the joy you experience when you accomplish more than you ever dreamed possible. Being with a health coach or nutritionist is like having a support system with you at all times. You can do the DASH effect program without a health coach, or nutritionist, however, you cannot do it without an accountability partner. Their job is to keep you on track and then celebrate when you accomplish small victories until you reach the biggest accomplishment of your life.

An accountability partner is just that, a partner. Someone that stands with you in solidarity and supports your efforts to make positive changes in your life. If you hire a health coach, they have many useful tools to help you with your transformation while you're on the DASH effect diet. If you have an accountability partner that is just a friend or family member, their role in your journey is to support you, give you motivational pep talks, help you make proper choices, check in with you often to see how it's going, and also remind you of why you are making these changes to your lifestyle.

Meal prep worksheet

When it comes to preparing your meal plan for the week, you should pick options from this list of allowable food items. You need a specific number of servings per food group for your daily intake of calories. Listed below is the amount of each item you need with options for that food group that is acceptable.

Pick the appropriate amount from each list and then arrange them in an easy-to-follow meal plan in the sections provided for each day of the week.

Grains (7 servings per day)	Meats (2-3 servings per day)
Vegetables (5 servings per day)	Nuts (2 servings per day)
Fruit (5 servings per day)	Fats (3 servings per day)
Dairy (3 servings per day)	Sweets (2 servings per week)

Permissible foods

Apples	Asparagus
Avocado	Broccoli
Berries (strawberries, blueberries)	Bell peppers (sweet)
Cantaloupe	Carrots
Cherries	Collard greens
Cherry tomatoes	Cucumbers
Celery	Dark green lettuce (not iceberg)
Grapefruit	Hot peppers
Grapes	Eggplant

Kiwi	Kale
Lemon	Red leafy lettuce
Mangoes	Spinach
Papayas	Summer squash
Peaches	Sweet corn
Pears	Sweet potato
Pineapple	Mushrooms
Tangerines	
Watermelon	
Chicken	Brown Rice
Catfish	Cereal
Cod	Whole-grain bread
Crab	Whole-wheat pasta
Egg whites	Almonds
Halibut	Lentils
Lean ground beef	Kidney beans
Shrimp	Peas
Tuna	Sunflower seeds
Turkey	
Salmon	
Low-fat mayonnaise	Fat-free milk
Margarine (no salt added)	Low-fat milk

Olive oil	Low-fat yogurt
Low-fat baked goods	Low-fat cheese
Low-fat jelly	Coffee (decaffeinated)
Low-fat sorbet	Tea (green)
Low-fat candies	Basil
Sugar treats	Bay leaf
	Cayenne
	Chive
	Cinnamon
	Clove
	Endive
	Garlic
	Ginger
	Mint
	Parsley
	Pepper
	Rosemary
	Sage
	Turmeric

Meal prep weekly plan

Example meal prep weekly plan

Monday	Ingredients
Breakfast: • Fresh mixed fruits, (1 cup) • Bran muffin (1) • Trans-free margarine (1 teaspoon) • Fat-free milk (1 cup) • Herbal tea	• melons, banana, apple, and berries • topped with fat-free, low-calorie vanilla-flavored yogurt (1 cup) • Walnuts (0.33 cup)
Lunch: • Spinach salad made with: reduced-sodium wheat crackers (12) • Fat-free milk (1 cup)	• Fresh spinach leaves (4 Cups) • Slivered almonds (0.33 cup) • Sliced pear (1) • Canned mandarin orange sections (0.50 cup) • Red wine vinaigrette (2 Tablespoons)

Dinner:	Kabob made with:
<ul><li>Beef and vegetable kebab,</li><li>Pecans (0.33 cup)</li><li>Cooked wild rice (1 cup)</li><li>Pineapple chunks (1 cup)</li><li>Cran-Raspberry spritzer</li></ul>	<ul><li>Peppers, mushrooms and onions, cherry tomatoes (1 cup each)</li><li>Beef (3 ounces)</li><li>Spritzer made with: sparkling water (4-8 ounces)</li><li>Cran-Raspberry juice (4 ounces)</li></ul>

Monday	Ingredients
Breakfast	
Lunch	
Dinner	

Tuesday	Ingredients
Breakfast	
Lunch	
Dinner	

Wednesday	Ingredients
Breakfast	
Lunch	
Dinner	

Thursday	Ingredients
Breakfast	
Lunch	
Dinner	

Friday	Ingredients
Breakfast	
Lunch	
Dinner	

Saturday	Ingredients
Breakfast	
Lunch	
Dinner	

Sunday	Ingredients
Breakfast	
Lunch	
Dinner	

As you can see at the top of the meal preparation worksheet, I have included a sample of meal preparation. When planning meals for the day or week, it is best to put them on paper so you can see in detail exactly what you want to have and what ingredients you need. By preparing this in advance, you are taking a lot of the guesswork out of meal preparations. Earlier in the book, we discussed how knowing what you need at the grocery store helps you prepare for your meals without overspending at the grocery store. Being proactive with your meal preparations helps budget your grocery bill. For instance, when you go to the grocery store, you are not going to buy a bunch of stuff that you don't need if you already made a list of the groceries you need for the DASH effect diet program.

Each section represents a day in the week, and each block within that table is designated for meal time. Within each mealtime, you should list the name or type of meal it is, e.g. 'Slow cooked chicken.' Then on the right-hand side is the section where you list your ingredients. This will not only help in preparing the meal when the time comes, but it will also provide you with a grocery list for each week's combined meal plans. By writing this out, you are better preparing yourself for a healthier lifestyle. You can utilize this same process for every week. If you want to be a bit more proactive, you can plan your meals for several weeks out.

Some people prepare a whole meal plan for a month, as this helps them organize their weeks and days better, as well as budget their grocery shopping. By meal planning with a detailed diagram such as this one, you can make sure that you won't be eating the same meals every week as well. This gives you more options for variety in your food preparations and also allows you to see your week's meal preparation in an organized fashion, helping you eliminate the need to hunt and find something to prepare for the evening.

One thing to remember is to prepare enough that you can save your leftovers for the next day or two to save on grocery money. For instance, if you make cinnamon apples for your night time snack or if you decided on having fruit for dinner, you can blend the leftovers together and make applesauce for your morning oats tomorrow. Many of the dishes you can make for dinner can be utilized for lunch the next day, eliminating the need to prepare a designated meal plan for every single day. It also allows you to cut down on your food expenses by giving you two meals out of one grocery purchase.

If you are a single serving household, you may even get several meals out of each recipe that you make. If you prepare a meal that can serve four people, that should allow you to have lunch for the next day and dinner for the day after that. Remember, food stays fresh if it's frozen after being cooked. So, if you prepare a larger meal and only need one serving at a time,

66

freezing the remaining portions is a great way to extend your meals for more than one day or week.

If you can squeeze in enough time, you may even prep all weekly meals in one day of the week like Sunday for example. Then you freeze them in containers and pull them out as needed. If you only need one serving of each item per meal, then you must remember to only store it in single serving sections so that you are not reheating the excess and potentially ruin the possibility of having that meal on another day. Since reheating can spoil food if it's frozen and reheated again, you should only reheat what you're going to eat.

Calorie intake tracking worksheet

For each meal you prepare, you want to keep track of the calories that you are taking in. This includes all nutritional values. This is not to keep track of calories, but it's more about keeping track of your progress with the DASH effect diet plan. This is a simple process that can easily be done by using the packaging from your food choices to record the nutritional calorie intake from the serving size suggested on the package.

If you use fresh vegetables and fruits, this can be a little bit tricky. So I am listing a few of them below so you can have a few clues as to what you would need to write down for those fresh fruits and vegetables while you're on the DASH effect diet. You can find these nutritional statistics online at the FDA website. Once you have a guideline for fresh fruits and vegetables, record that data and utilize it to meet the conditions on your calorie tracker.

Servings sizes per fruit or vegetable

A vegetable's serving size is one cup of raw mixed greens or 0.50 cup of chopped vegetables. A fruit's serving size is 1 medium fruit or a 0.50 cup of fresh, frozen, or canned fruit:

Apples

- Calories 130

- Potassium 260mg

- Total carbohydrates 34g

- Dietary fiber 5g

- Sugars 25g

- Proteins 1g

Bananas

- Calorie 110

- Potassium 450mg

- Total carbohydrates 30g

- Dietary fiber 3g

- Sugars 19g

- Protein 1g

Grapes

- Calories 90

- Sodium 15mg

- Potassium 240mg

- Total carbohydrates 23g

- Dietary fiber 1g

- Sugars 20g

Pineapple

- Calories 50

- Sodium 10mg

- Potassium 120mg

- Total carbohydrates 13g

- Dietary fiber 1g

- Sugar 10g protein 1g

Asparagus

- Calories 20

- Potassium 230mg

- Total carbohydrates 4g

- Dietary fiber 2g

- Sugar 2g

- Protein 2g

Carrot

- Calories 30

- Sodium 60mg

- Potassium 250mg

- Total carbohydrates 7g

- Dietary fiber 2g

- Sugars 5g

- Proteins 1g

Mushrooms

- Calories 20

- Sodium 15mg

- Potassium 300mg

- Total carbohydrates 3g

- Dietary Fiber 1g

- Protein 3g

So, as you can see, you will list the nutrients that are shown here. Most of the time you will have sodium, potassium, total carbohydrates, dietary fiber, sugar, and protein on the list. These things are what you would add together to find your total intake of those nutrients. The calories section is a combined rating of these nutrients, and that is what you will need to add together to get the total daily calorie intake to meet the 2000 calories recommended by the USDA.

At the bottom of the tracker worksheets, there is an example you can utilize for your calorie tracking needs. Each meal is labeled at the top as breakfast, lunch, dinner, and snack or drink. This helps you know exactly which column to put the calories and nutrients under. The side column has listings for several of the nutrients that you want to keep track of. If you notice at the top of the chart, that is the total calories for that meal. At the end of the day, you can add all the calories together to make sure you actually had the proper intake of calories for a full day. The average calorie intake is 2,000 calories depending on your size, age, and activity level.

Calories and nutrients tracker

Nutritional Data Monday	Breakfast	Lunch	Dinner	Snack and drinks
Calories				
Potassium				
Total Carbohydrates				
Dietary fiber				
Sugar				
Protein				
sodium				

Nutritional Data Tuesday	Breakfast	Lunch	Dinner	Snack and drinks
Calories				
Potassium				
Total Carbohydrates				
Dietary fiber				
Sugar				
Protein				
sodium				

Nutritional Data Wednesday	Breakfast	Lunch	Dinner	Snack and drinks
Calories				
Potassium				
Total Carbohydrates				
Dietary fiber				
Sugar				
Protein				
sodium				

Nutritional Data Thursday	Breakfast	Lunch	Dinner	Snack and drinks
Calories				
Potassium				
Total Carbohydrates				
Dietary fiber				
Sugar				
Protein				
sodium				

Nutritional Data Friday	Breakfast	Lunch	Dinner	Snack and drinks
Calories				
Potassium				
Total Carbohydrates				
Dietary fiber				
Sugar				
Protein				
sodium				

Nutritional Data Saturday	Breakfast	Lunch	Dinner	Snack and drinks
Calories				
Potassium				
Total Carbohydrates				
Dietary fiber				
Sugar				
Protein				
sodium				

Nutritional Data Sunday	Breakfast	Lunch	Dinner	Snack and drinks
Calories				
Potassium				
Total Carbohydrates				
Dietary fiber				
Sugar				
Protein				
sodium				

Example of the nutrition tracker

Nutritional Data Sunday	Breakfast	Lunch	Dinner	Snack and drinks
Calories	252	194	251	150
Potassium	822mg	410mg	894mg	119mg
Total Carbohydrates	33g	27g	2g	27g
Dietary fiber	8g	4g	less than 1g	1g
Sugar	8g	1g	less than 1g	9g
Protein	11g	17g	34g	3g
sodium	102mg	450mg	78mg	52mg

After a week of tracking what your calorie intake is, you will be able to see where you need to adjust your diet and how to make it less sodium-heavy and more protein, potassium, magnesium, and calcium heavy. Our health is determined by what we choose to eat. If you chose to eat fatty and greasy foods, then your body will become sluggish, tired, weak, and you might end up suffering from hypertension, diabetes, and sometimes heart conditions.

Conclusion

Thank you for making it through to the end of *The DASH Effect: Instantly Return Your Body to Peak Physical Form*, I hope it was informative and that it provided you with all of the tools you need to achieve your goal of attaining better health with the DASH effect diet. Now that you have read all there is to know about the DASH effect, you should be ready to start your journey where you will have a life without hypertension, diabetes, cancer, excess weight, and so many other diseases that plague us.

The next step in this process is to talk to your doctor about any concerns you may have, which I hope are not many. Then look into finding an accountability partner or health coach. Once you have determined which process you will use with your support system, you are almost at the finish line. Make a conscious effort to plan a week's worth of meals that will incorporate all that you have learned in this book and then get busy eliminating the bad foods that are already in your pantry. Once you have made room for new groceries, it's time to go to the store and pick up the new foods that you will need.

One thing you can do to help ensure that you are not going to fall back into your old habits is to remove the things which might trigger you. So throw out your salt, eliminate the processed foods that are not good for you, replace your canned goods with fresh vegetables and fruits, and above all, remember that this is not rocket science. It is a simple eating plan based on clean, fresh ingredients and reduced consumption of sodium.

Do not be discouraged if you fail every now and then. You don't have to derail your entire plan to start all over again if you do. Just remind yourself that you are only human and as a human, we sometimes make mistakes. I hope that with the help of this book you found the answers you needed and hopefully, you can teach others about the benefits of the DASH effect diet.